HOLY SH*T,
MY KID IS CUTTING!

THE COMPLETE PLAN
TO STOP SELF HARM

BY J.J. KELLY, Psy.D.

HOLY SH*T, MY KID IS CUTTING!

THE COMPLETE PLAN TO STOP SELF-HARM

Difference Press, Washington, D.C., USA

ISBN: 978-1-68309-245-2

Cover Design: Jennifer Stimson
Editing: Moriah Howell
Author's photo courtesy of Melissa Schmidt of Icarian Photography

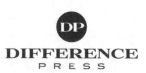

DIFFERENCE
PRESS

For Joey P.
Thank you for always reminding me to
"Live the Question."

TABLE OF CONTENTS

CHAPTER 1
VALIDATING "SCARY"

I had just hosted the first Young Women's Empowerment Group — or, that's what I called it — in my home. There were seven young women ages nineteen to thirty sitting in my living room. One I'd worked with for about a year, some I met five years ago…a couple of them, almost ten years ago. When I met them, several were cutting themselves, a few punching walls 'til their knuckles bloodied. There had to be at least ten serious suicide attempts between the seven of them. A couple had been fairly catatonic; one had beaten her own face so swollen on one side before she came into our second session that I had to send her to the ER immediately. A couple were on a suicidal path with booze, several had spent serious time inpatient and institutionalized, and I'd put money on every single one of them thinking of taking their own life more than a couple of times.

Jesus.

As I write this, I think of you, a terrified parent... wanting — well, actually, needing help. You need help now.

You discovered your kid is cutting. The person you made is actually hurting themselves on purpose. The questions go on and on and on: "Why would anyone do that? Why would my kid do that? What is going on with them? What are they not telling me? Do they want to die?"

First of all, let me just say I get it. This is so scary. There is something so against nature that a human being would want to hurt themselves on purpose.

But those young women at my Empowerment Group are the most emotionally intelligent people I have met, and I've trained with geniuses. But even geniuses with letters after their names don't have the emotional aware-ness and vocabulary, the ego-strength and resilience, the generosity and ability to empathically and actively listen that these few young women have – they don't. These skills can only develop from finding the courage to explore oneself fully, honestly. You can only get this good at expressing your emotions and thoughts and beliefs and dreams from one thing…and these women have it.

They like themselves.

They have worked their asses off – many of them for years – to learn who they are and accept themselves, flaws and all. They have found themselves on the other side of the tunnel where they genuinely hold themselves in self-re-spect and self-love. Not the kind on t-shirts sold in yoga studios. The real deal. They have learned to like them-selves. They are the kind of people that are in a crowd of black and white and they shine with color. And I have had the privilege of teaching them. I am so happy, and I am so deeply proud of them all. I'm excited for their future and the impact they can now have on the world – now that they have freed themselves from the ignorance that is required to hate, or even dislike yourself.

I didn't cure them. I just taught them the skills to effectively manage their emotions so they can find who they really are and what their values are so they can act according to those values and reinforce their self-esteem and self-confidence. Because that's what I believe: global healing can be achieved by teaching people how to like themselves.

And for me, that starts one kid at a time. That includes your kid.

You have felt the terror that comes with learning your kid is cutting. If you came into my office for a first appointment, I would likely introduce myself, offer you tea, follow you into the room, and gesture for you to have a seat on the couch. I'd then sit across from you and likely say, "So what's goin' on?"

You'd probably be nervous, but launch into it anyway. We'd spend the next twenty to thirty minutes with you telling me about how shocked you are to find out your kid is hurting themselves on purpose, and how you feel sad because they used to be so happy and active and they used to talk to you, but not anymore. You'd say how you feel guilty because you thought their moodiness was just a teenager thing and you had no idea how serious this was.

I probably wouldn't say much – I'm sure I'd be emphatically nodding the whole time you expressed your feelings, probably adding several times, "Totally. Yep. Totally. Super scary, yeah" and you'd feel comforted… and calmer, because you'd know I meant it. I'd actively listen, not taking my eyes from you at all while you talked, taking in all of what you were saying. I wouldn't interrupt you. You'd have minutes of a slow and concerned cadence, and then as your worry increased with the details you told me, you'd speed up and get a bit louder. I'd stay out of your way and let you tell me your story, until you came to a pause where you probably wouldn't yet ask me out loud, but you'd look at me with the question in your eyes, "So what do you think I should do?" And then we'd get into it. I'd start off, "So, this is what I'm thinking…" I'd let you know that I get what you're going through, I really do. I have seen that pained look on the faces of many parents, and heard it in the voices of many, many more. I would easily and authentically validate your fear, your sadness, your guilt. And I'd let you know how many times I've seen this before and how many times kids have pulled out of it to become healthy and happy young adults and adults. And so it begins… except what I do is have that same first meeting with your kid. When a kid is cutting, parents and professionals send them to me.

CHAPTER 2
TEEN WHISPERER

I have no idea what the literal count is, but I've seen hundreds of kids – and I wouldn't be at all surprised if it's in the thousands. When I say "kids," I mean pretty much anyone under thirty – certainly twenty-five because the brain isn't even fully formed yet. Saying kid takes care of gender pronouns and age determination, which adds a layer of privacy to the stories in this book. And I mean it endearingly. I call every one of the young people I work with kid…and they get it. So, anytime I say kid in this book, I mean your teenager or grown child: ages fifteen to twenty-six-ish.

Even back in the early 2000s, when I was an intern, I got these kids. I think it started just because supervisors thought I was energetic and pretty mouthy and I might be able to handle teenagers. Which is how I have come to learn that many shrinks (I use *this* term generally for anyone with a doctoral level education in psych; so, psychologists and psychiatrists alike, although they are *nothing* alike, but we'll get to that later) are actually afraid to work with teenagers. I certainly have my own theories on *that*. But I also definitely got these referrals because interns are cheap (meaning inexpensive) and I was an intern.

So, I was lucky enough to get trained by some super-smarty-pantses — very well-educated veterans in the field — psychologists, psychiatrists, MFTs (marriage and family therapists), neuropsychologists...really, some of the best around. The place was established the year before I was born, and I was the first one to be offered a staff position in decades, I think. As I was coming up, I was seen as a go-getter who would take any case referred to me, and I now know that finding a low-cost trainee that is competent is no small feat. Hell, finding a full-fledged licensed psychologist that's competent is an accomplishment, in my opinion. I mean, think about *why* people go into mental health. It doesn't take letters after your name to deduce that it's probably because of some unresolved emotional issues from childhood that we wanted to figure out in undergrad and just kept going. Problem is, giving advice is not the same as listening. Thinking you're "right" and using fancy psych terms to intellectually justify your opinion are definitely not the same as connecting. It's not *all* just problem solving; it's meeting the person in front of you where they are and learning how to help. So, while I'm not right in front of you listening to your sheer panic and sadness and guilt, I can easily validate you. And I know I can help.

I pretty quickly began to develop my knowledge and skill in dialectical behavior therapy, or DBT. DBT was originally developed by Dr. Marsha Lenihan for inpatient, chronically suicidal people with a borderline personality disorder (BPD) diagnosis. And how many of those do you suppose are women? Yeah, the vast majority – big surprise to find out women are both dismissed by medical doctors (psychiatrists) *and* over-pathologized. Here's another news flash, too: when people are struggling and they don't get decent mental health providers, they tend to get worse. So, as self-harm is a very common symptom of BPD, and DBT was gathering steam in effectiveness treating BPD. *Voila!* I was getting a ton of referrals for people engaging in self-harm behaviors – most commonly cutting.

The psychiatrists (both in my group practice and in the Berkeley/Bay Area community) often referred kids to me – despite ageism, narcissism, and sexism in the field and society in general – when they had no idea what to do with their patient/"this one," but masked it with the air of "I'm doing you a huge favor." They'd also hint about not expecting me to get anywhere with the kid, but I probably couldn't screw them up more. (Like adding more and more meds to the kids' daily regimen isn't tanking them already...psychiatrists are the worst. Yeah, I know – not *all* psychiatrists.)

While we're on the topic, I've stopped calling the people I work with "patients." The people that trained me operated under the medical model, and I've come to really disagree with that model. I don't believe that everyone who comes to me for help is "sick." I *do* think they're suffering and they don't know how to pull themselves out of it, and it's no wonder. Where did you learn in elementary school, high school, or college about how to effectively manage emotions? Yeah, nowhere. What I find is that, unlike the medical model that roots out symptoms and treats those symptoms, most people have resilience and reserves of strength that can be tapped in times of intense emotions and crisis. I also see, time and time again, that when I expect strength and an ability to tolerate pain, that's exactly what I get. When doctors expect only pathology and maladaptive symptoms from their "patients," that's usually what they get. I think that's backward, and it robs people of the self-confidence points that come from weathering something difficult and scary. Inviting people to find the courage to trust themselves and use their skills builds empowerment. So, I call people who work with me *participants* because I demand so much courage and work from them that they deserve a more active descriptor. These kids really work hard.

So, here's the thing: the kids who have worked with me slowed down their self-harm behaviors. And then they *stopped* cutting. Over and over again, these kids, who often had a long history of cutting, depression, tanking grades, withdrawal from friends…we'd see their spark come back. I could see them smiling a little more. We'd laugh together a bit more in our work. They'd have more energy in their faces and in how they walked – even their posture and eye contact improved. And lemme tell ya… when the light comes back on in the face of kid who's been down awhile, sometimes even a *long* while, it is a thrilling thing. I think the pilot light was still on in their heart and brain, but they've been so progressively unhappy, they got lost in it and needed some guidance to get back (or forward) to themselves. And then they could soar.

Clinically, I have seen kids in really dark places...so dark it scares parents to death. And cutting has a weird secrecy around it that no one really has words for – regular words that help us all really understand, not just medical words that make a doctor look smarter. I go looking for the kid. I listen, like, *really* listen to what they have to say about it and many other things, like music and video games, their friends, their clothes, memes...y'know, the stuff that's important when you're that age. You remember, right? Yeah, that's the thing: Teenagers and young adults believe they are chronically dismissed by adults. I happen to agree with that. As a society, we do dismiss them. We blow off what young people have to say. They don't have the experience in life to have built credibility like adults, so they're treated more like children, which they also definitely are not. Yet, what I see more and more is that though they're not taken seriously for their ideas, they *are* held to responsibilities – especially around academic achievements – that are definitely more pressure than anyone should put on a kid. Also, with the politics of today being in the forefront, they have way more grown-up worries than they used to bear, but the same amount of dismissal and lack of voice as before. These kids are stressed. They are self-harming in all kinds of ways...including cutting.

The last reason I think I've been so successful in treating kids that hurt themselves is because, as you've probably guessed, when I was young, I dabbled in cutting myself. No one ever caught me, but I remember the intense emotions I had as a young person. I remember having no real tools to cope with all those really strong emotions. And I didn't tell anyone, so I was alone with it. It sucked. And now I can use that to help young people learn tools to cope with *anything* they're feeling. And they can use those tools *instead* of cutting. And instead of feeling the sadness and shame that self-harm brings, they can feel proud of themselves for choosing the healthy alternatives that I teach them. I actually am grateful for that turbulent time, because now I have this deep understanding of pain – self- and other-inflicted. I have had the profound privilege of using that knowledge to help kids of all ages not only *stop* hurting themselves, but *start* liking themselves enough to know they deserve healthy alternatives to coping with life.

CHAPTER 3
TOO LATE TO WAIT

I have definitely seen some gnarly stuff in the last fifteen years of treating cutting and other self-harm behaviors. Though I believe and have *seen* the vast majority of kids recover and thrive, I want you to know and be *really* clear on one hard fact: cutting does *not* go away on its own. You really do have to address this now that you're aware of it. I have seen those parents who, for whatever reason, try to ignore self-harm behaviors. I assume they feel fear and that leads to their denial. They're not terrible people. It's really easy for me to validate a parent's fear and their impulse to ignore it and hope everything'll just get better. Shit, we all have impulses to do that sometimes when a crisis arises. I validate the *impulses* to avoid, not the *behavior* of avoiding. We, as humans, may want to run away from scary things, but rational, intelligent people know that is not always the wisest thing to do. And I strongly suggest you find your courage and use your rational, logical mind on this one because this is a crisis point for your kid.

The emotions causing distress are leaking out now, beyond containment and management. You literally have physical evidence of your kid's emotional pain on their body. A nineteen-year-old said to me the other day, "If I'd had a broken arm they wouldn't have ignored it and waited to get me to a doctor, but because they couldn't *see* the twist in my brain they didn't get me a doctor's help. But they knew I wasn't ok." That's heart-wrenching, right? And this kid's parents aren't monsters. They just don't have the emotional intelligence to understand what's going on with their kid. How *would* they? Where are we taught that? When was the lesson in school on naming and managing emotions? Who encourages us, as a society, to prioritize learning to name and manage emotions to increase the quality of our *lives!?*

Seeking psychological help is still stigmatized as crazy and medicalized through a pharmaceutical lens, and it costs money that more and more is not subsidized by governmental help. I'll tell you this much, though, it's gonna cost you a helluva lot more money if your kid is cutting now and you wait on getting help and things go downhill. Then we're talking wilderness programs, therapeutic boarding schools, hospitalization, jail and/or lawyers, failing/dropping out of college, detox programs, and/or other inpatient programs. I don't want to terrify you, I just want to impress upon you the importance of facing this head-on, and not to wait and see on it. Having a distant or strained relationship with your kid in their twenties and thirties may not cost as much as treatment for cutting, but that's only in terms of money.

So here's what we're going to do – I'm going to give you everything I know about cutting and self-harm. All angles. I'm going to deliver it in a way I think you can digest without overwhelm. Since a calmer brain operates more efficiently, I'm going to help you wrap your head around your fear in Chapter 4 so you can learn some important distinctions between self-medication (Chapter 5) and medication management (Chapter 7). I'll help you explore the stressors that are most likely contributing to your kid's self-harm in Chapter 6 and how to ride out the bumps that come with change (Chapter 8). Once you get some of that knowledge under your belt, you'll be equipped for the importance of Chapter 9, which outlines how to choose a professional to work with your kid. Then in Chapter 10, we'll build the concrete home plan to support the end of self-harm in your family.

Hang in there. I know you'll feel calmer and more powerfully equipped to effectively deal with your kid's cutting by the end of this book. Truly. Knowledge is power.

CHAPTER 4
DON'T FREAK

So don't freak out. I mean, do – for a minute. Ok, freak out and simultaneously tell yourself this problem is *temporary*. In my clinical opinion, you've already taken the important and most difficult step. The step from doing *nothing* to doing *something*. The hardest one is over. You're not in denial – or maybe some but not enough that you're flat-out ignoring the problem. You've accepted the reality that this is happening and you do need to act and get your kid some help to stop cutting. Way to not go "rag doll" or "possum," as I call it. Passivity is the worst choice to make right now, and you've already chosen action, so *kudos!*

Yes, you're scared because *it's scary*. I am not here to talk you out of that. In general, I think people believe that helping means meeting the person where they are and helping them solve the problem. Yes. Conceptually. Theoretically, people know that. But who the hell *does* that!? How many times have you come home from a crappy day at work, put down your bag, and started to tell your partner about what a tyrant your boss was today, and the *first* thing out of their mouth is, "Well, maybe what she *meant* was"!? Or you're out for a drink with co-workers and same thing: you have a boss complaint and another co-worker says, "Well when he said that to *me*, I just…" Or how about you complain about your partner to a close friend and they respond, "Well, at least they don't do [some bullshit thing *their* partner does and now the conversation is about them]"!? It sucks. It's a "miss" of meeting you where you are *first*. And therapists do this unhelpful garbage, too.

You may be thinking I'm doing it right now – you're scared and I'm going to write this chapter telling you all the reasons you don't need to be. Nope. The difference is I *validated* your fear *first*. And I'll help you *through* it, not try to convince you shouldn't feel it.

Once again for the nosebleed section: *Validation has to come before problem solving.* I cannot emphasize enough how important this practice is, and I do it every day. I teach it every day. The reason people who actually *want* to help constantly "miss" and jump to problem solving is because they are anxious about your discomfort and don't manage their anxiety effectively (because where would they have learned that?) and unconsciously make the whole interaction about *them* and getting rid of their anxiety by accidentally telling you to get rid of yours. Like that's ever, in the history of humans, worked. On *top* of making it about them, it's also unsolicited advice, which we know everyone loves right?

No.

When you were venting about your boss, did you *ask* for a solution from your work friend? Did you ever once say, "Hey, Cheryl, I bet you've had this happen and I bet you handled it better than anything *I'd* ever think of, so tell me what to do." No. Nope. Clinically, it is my solemn wish that *everyone* would eliminate words/phrases like:

- "Should/shouldn't"
- "Well, actually..." (the mansplainers' fave)
- "At least..." (never not *invalidating*)
- "Well, not only *that*..." (code for: I didn't even listen to your point, I was just waiting to talk)

And the thing is, I'm a psychologist, so the "solicited advice" thing is built in, but I *still* don't talk to people like this because it's not effective for active listening. Plus, I just think it's rude. I think these phrases are used by people with no skill for listening, people whose objective is to make the conversation about themselves as soon as they can, people who feel insecure and go around trying to prove how many facts they know while demonstrating how little they know about human connection and joy. Narcissism is an epidemic, People!...but that's another book.

You're going to need the skill of validation for dealing with your kid throughout this process of recovery from self-harm. So, breathe, and let me give you a couple of pointers:

1. You need not *agree* with someone in order to properly validate them. For instance, when I'm working with someone who appears to be getting

in their own way, I'm not going to say, "That's an excellent point, she *does* suck," if I don't agree. I might say something more accurate like, "I can see she pissed you off." Then, I'm joining the person where they are without violating my own values of honesty. The more truthful example connects us without reducing authenticity. Get it? *You* think of one now, specific to your life; actual events that happened recently are the most effective ones. Example: if your fifteen-year-old daughter gets in the car after school and immediately says she's never talking to a friend she's had since fourth grade ever again, it may be very tempting to point out how she seems to be friends and then not be friends with other girls every other week – not to mention the constant use of hyperbole. I often just laugh out loud, but I'm fairly certain you'd get skewered for the exact same thing. But even if you meet your daughter with something much more tempered and reasonable like, "Well, honey, you've been friends with her since you two were little…I'm sure you'll work it out." You've engaged in a missed connection with your daughter. She will experience the first part as wholly invalidating and the second half as problem solving without "getting it." I'm not even remotely saying I'd disagree with your assessment of the situation, I just know your daughter, as a result of this realistic sentence, will tell you less. On the other hand, a simple, "Oh no? What happened?"

and then listening without interruption or advice will open the door and *keep* it open.

2. Discipline yourself to language your validation statements using *"and,"* never *"but."* If I say, "You look so sad, but…" What the hell could I possibly say next that would go well? Any time a "but" follows a validation statement, it *invalidates* the validation statement. Everybody knows this *but* still does it. See what I did there!? How about, "Everybody knows this *and* still does it"? Look – the "but" in the first sentence nicely illustrates how everybody must *not* know it or they wouldn't do it. I think you'll be surprised the impact this little tweak will have. When you discipline yourself to say, "I hear what you're saying, *and…*" and you mean it, you *did* listen to them when they were making their point, *even* if you disagree you increase your chances of a smoother interpersonal interaction by not invalidating them. All my participants (many are young) train themselves to speak in this way *and* you can do it, too.

While we're in the groove of validating your fear about your kid cutting, let's take a look at how often cutting occurs. First of all, the research on cutting is sparse and contradictory. Most studies examine the more broad category of NSSI (nonsuicidal self-injury), but a lot of data is about inpatient residents. There has been almost no research done on NSSI in youth of color, which is abysmally typical, but it is worth noting that Native

American youth may have the highest incidence of NSSI. This supports my belief that cutting and self-harm are symptoms of trauma.

I wanted to find numbers to put your mind at ease that this thing has an end, but since the data appears incomplete, inconclusive, and biased, let me just level with you about what I see and have seen:

- Most studies agree that the most common NSSI is cutting.

- Many studies say up to half of adolescents (not a lot of age breakdowns) self-harm. I'd say that number is close, though low.

- Females seem to cut themselves more, but males punch things more – gender politics seem to be at play, though no studies I saw discussed the over-pathologizing of women and people of color, or that the only socially-sanctioned emotions for males to express is anger.

- While ignored self-harm behaviors get worse if not treated professionally, in my opinion, they do seem to drop off around twenty-four years old, often with another maladaptive coping strategy taking its place.

And I have no clue what the stats are regarding my own practice. What I will tell you, though, is that kids who work with me turn it around. The ones who can hang with my style (and it is not for everyone, to be sure) and stick, they do brave and important and difficult work with me. And I have the great pleasure of watching them save their own lives in my office. Best job ever. I really cannot say enough about the courage of the kids I've worked with. They find strength within themselves they were sure they never had. Your kid can do that, too. Really, they can.

CHAPTER 5
SELF-MEDICATION

We humans are animals. I think we often forget that because we spend so much time in our heads. I remember reading a stat that we have eighty-four percent identical DNA to a mouse. A mouse! It's in the high nineties with orangutans. Even if you've read those stats and you accept them as fact, we often forget to look at our behaviors and our experiences through that lens. We forget, in our daily lives, that we are genetically wired for fear. Fear is our prominent survival tactic, and the fear instinct is so strong that we often make our decisions in reaction to it.

There's more and more talk about humans' wiring for fear, but it appears we are not also shedding our shame when we feel fear. Why is that? That our socialization as humans dictates that we must feel shame for an emotional experience that is instinctual and has kept us alive for what, six million years? Why, then, with this widely accepted truth that fear is natural, do we have so little practical knowledge about how to effectively manage it? And why, as an American society, do we put so little value on learning about our emotions and learning tools to effectively manage our emotions as to increase our quality of life and our capacity to experience joy? After all, isn't *that* what it's supposed to be all about!? Perhaps it's a philosophical question, although I think it's basically because someone benefits from our collective ignorance – and, therefore, it's more of a socio-political one (and there's another book). What I have seen, clinically, is that most people who have not been taught to manage their emotions effectively do one of a handful of things:

1. They attempt to convince themselves their emotions are not really happening, and everything is "fine."

2. They project their emotions out onto something, or usually some*one* else, most likely in the form of criticism. In the car: "That asshole cut me off on purpose!" You thought the car pulling in front of you might collide with you, which kicked in your fight or flight response to perceived imminent harm or death, you have not been taught the tools to manage fear effectively, so the fear get projected out as criticism – a narrative about how that person cut you off "on purpose," which reflects that they are a "bad person." Wow. All just a made-up story. Fear is, indeed, a liar.

3. They try to find a way to control their environment, including other people, in order to "predict" the future so they won't be "caught off

guard," which is both driven by *and* causes more fear.

4. Find a way not to feel.

The tendency to make our world into "black or white," "right or wrong," "worthwhile or worthless" is rampant and is linked to high rates of anxiety and depression. So why do people do it, then? Well:

1. We're hard-wired for fear.

2. We do not get taught tools to effectively name, accept, and manage fear.

When I work with participants (remember, I don't say "patients") of any age, I talk about the acceptance of living in the gray – and it's *all* gray. I challenge people to accept that all reality is gray, and instead of clinging to a manufactured concept of "certainty," perhaps it would be more effective to learn how to manage the anxiety that naturally comes from the "I don't know." That we're all just bumbling around in life, making our best educated guess about everything...and that's ok. Yeah, that takes time and a *lot* of hard work and conversation and *listening* to each other. And while we're doing this existential-level work, we also need to accurately identify how we currently self-medicate our emotions until we have those tools to manage them head-on.

Self-medication is *not* taking an ibuprofen for a headache. Self-medication methods are the behaviors we humans engage in *instead* of dealing with our emotions. All four of those sets of behaviors previously mentioned above are ways people self-medicate. We avoid, we try to control, we push down, we deny, we off-load onto some-one else *all* the emotions we don't have tools for. Espe-cially fear, since that's the emotion most humans experi-ence most frequently.

Since at its core it is a behavior meant to avoid emo-tions, self-medication is not healthy. And the kinds of self-medicating behaviors we see in modern humans are, strangely, widely accepted and socially normalized. Behaviors like imbibing in:

- Alcohol
- Tobacco
- Benzos – to slow down (e.g., Valium, Xanax, Ativan)
- Speed – including caffeine and prescriptions like Adderall and Ritalin
- Weed

These are all actual substances, but self-medication comes in other forms that are also harmful:

- Workaholism
- Internet browsing/Netflix "binges"
- Working out
- Food – overeating, emotional eating, excess salt, sugar, fat, etc.

There are many more. And you'll notice that this is a mostly list of legal purchases aside from marijuana (not everywhere, yet), and, unless you have a prescription, benzos and most speed. Also, I have found the amount of high functioning adult professionals that mix benzos and wine shocks me. How many famous people have to die from this and other downer-downer combos? I'm alarmist about almost nothing, but benzos and alcohol consumed together (often casually) raises my eyebrows.

It's strange how using substances and over-relying on them is often only seen as a problem when it is illegal or puts someone into crisis, like:

- Cocaine

- Oxy

- Cutting

- Fatal extreme sport accidents – but non-fatal accidents are "cool"? And running marathons – though generally agreed upon is quite hard on the body – is societally viewed as a "high achievement" of a "highly disciplined" individual. The reality of what I see is that multiple marathoners are often actually "running away" from fear.

It's hard to know where society draws the line on where these behaviors lie – in the healthy or unhealthy camp. In psychology, an unhealthy or "maladaptive" behavior is often defined by if your involvement in the behavior is negatively impacting your ability to function at work, school, or in your social relationships. Ok, and who defines that? Now, I'm not saying there's a lot of interpretation or wiggle room in defining if cutting is healthy or unhealthy. Even people who cut themselves believe it is unhealthy to deliberately hurt themselves. But they do it because it works, meaning it reduces the intensity of the negative emotions that are currently overwhelming them and causing distress. They wouldn't do it if it didn't work. And in that way, cutting is much like problem drinking, or sex addiction, or any drug at all taken to numb-out a distressing emotion. And that can even be when that drug is prescribed.

So, in that way, I would argue that basically every human has engaged in self-harm behavior in one form or another likely many times in their lives. What if the routine of coming home from work and having a cocktail was, instead, a short neighborhood walk before dinner? Meditation, when practiced with some regularity, has been shown to lower blood pressure, heartrate and reduces inflammation. A martial art teaches a practice of disciplining the mind and using the body in a way one can defend themselves. Never underestimate the calming effect controlled hitting of something can have on raging adolescent hormones. I'd argue it's healthier (and more legal) than fighting with other humans, more active than escaping into video games, and definitely more compassionate than cyberbullying. I've seen a martial art build self-confidence in many people because mastery of a skillset and having the positive regard for one's self to believe we are worth defending often leads to a reduction and extinction of self-harm behaviors. And if we *taught* skills and tools for effectively regulating emotions – like as part of regular junior high or high school curriculum – I argue that we would be able to largely do away with *The Diagnostic & Statistical Manual of Mental Disorders* (that is foundationally biased) and most mental health disorders altogether. Very little research could reveal to you the groups that make these diagnoses, as well as the groups largely suffering from them – and how that reflects the power dynamics in this country and the world. By no means do you have to agree with me on this point. It is relevant to see cutting and other self-harm behaviors like fighting and food-restricting through the frame of self-medication because that is how we treat and eliminate cutting from your kid's coping répertoire. We've *got* to figure out what is causing such intense emotions in your kid that they arc unable to cope without hurting themselves. And we'll start to figure that out in the next chapter.

CHAPTER 6
FIND WHAT'S HIDING

Just stop and think, for a moment, what your high school experience was like. Were you in sports or clubs? What extracurriculars were your favorite? How were your grades? Did you have a solid group of friends? How'd you get along with your parents? What kinds of things did you do that they (your parents) didn't know about? Were you happy? If yes, what kinds of things were what contributed to your happiness? If no, why? What was going on?

One of the things that I notice all the time is how parents of teens and young adults are shocked by their kid's behaviors – mostly the not-so-awesome ones. And when I ask them about their high school experiences, the parents weren't all angels either. Many of them got in some lightweight "trouble" as a teen and/or young adult, yet are shocked to discover their own kid lied about where they were, or who they were with, or got caught drinking or smoking pot, or picked a fight with their parents and are generally pissy most of the time.

Now, in *no way* am I saying cutting should be normalized like some of the other negative behaviors one might expect as a teen and young adult. Truly. I am just saying, take some time to try to remember how hard it was being that age, or what it might be like to be a teenager now, in this day and age. These kids are stressed out. I had no idea that so much of my job would be teaching people to lighten up and have some fun. I love that, but I thought it would be reigning them in more, not opening them up as much as I do. Whether it be age differences, regional differences, and/or other factors I'll get into, it appears that this generation of young adults has more opportunity, access, comforts, and a whole lot more worries.

The differences in generations aren't as important, I don't think, unless we don't understand the difference in *stressors* of the generations. And, if your kid is cutting, something is definitely stressing your kid out past the point where they are equipped to handle it. Since not disclosing personal information to parents is somewhat of a teen and twenties hallmark of *any* generation, I'm going to tell you now; there's stuff you don't know. Let's get into that, so you can start to make educated guesses on what it might be, then you can sit down and ask your kid what's up with them. If they won't talk to you, you can guess and tell the clinician they will soon see. More on that later. For now, there are many areas of stress to consider with today's kids.

There are several stressors that I have discussed with teens and young adults over the last fifteen years that their parents initially did not know about or consider

when I started working with them. It's important to identify the factors that are causing distress in your kid's life
so we can figure out how to reduce their intensity and
manage the problem(s). The other reasons I want you
to consider each of these stressors, even the ones you're
"certain" have nothing to do with your kid, are because
I want you to practice finding your empathy. Imagine
what it might be like for you, if you were them- your
near-adult kid, if that stressor *was* their struggle. Then,
after you've found empathy for your kid inside each of
these imagined stressful situations, I want you to imagine
talking to your kid about what they're going through. In
this imagined interaction, I want you to imagine listening
without talking, waiting to talk, or offering problem-solv-
ing advice. Just listen to what your kid is telling you. Even
if what they're saying makes you anxious, just take three
deep breaths, don't interrupt, and keep listening. After
you've practiced this a bit, the "pro-move" as I call it,
what only the really emotionally intelligent participants
can do is to imagine and actually feel the gratitude that
comes from knowing you have cultivated a connection
and openness with your near-adult child that they are
the 1 in 1,000 of that age group that really *talks* to their
parents. Again, try this exercise with *each* of the following
stressors.

Grades

If your kid's grades have tanked recently, or are starting
to slip, there may be a few things to explain what's going
on here. Freshman year's a bitch. Whether it be the first

year of high school or the first year of college, I see a *ton* of struggling from kids who previously seemed "fine." Transitions are difficult for any of us, but both freshman years happen during biological, hormonal, and neuro-physiological changes, too. Puberty is in progress and the prefrontal cortex is not yet fully formed, which means the regulating emotions and processing information areas are in the trial and error phase and acting reactively or impulsively is prevalent. These biological changes of the human animal are to be considered when evaluating *all* these potential stressors, but especially in respect to grades and anxiety caused by the newness which are hallmarks of the freshman years. Often kids that were smart enough to skate by in junior high or middle school find that proper study habits are now a necessity in high school and they haven't developed any. Or, maybe they found the academics in high school a breeze and now they've entered college with very little discipline and/or time management skills and they're on their own now. It's hard to know what's going on – meaning, is it an emotional issue or something else?

This time period is often where kids get some testing at school or a neuropsychological evaluation to assess whether the student has some learning differences and/or emotional factors that negatively affect grades. I see a lot of UC-Berkeley first years come in having been valedictorian of their small high school, and find that their new pond is full of former big fish just like them. It blows their minds. It's in these kinds of instances where I see an influx of stimulants being prescribed to help the student "focus," and I would just strongly advise you *not* to put your kid on *any* form of speed without a neuropsych battery with someone with experience who's not afraid to say no to you. Long-term stimulant use by people who do not have ADHD/ADD can cause serious problems down the road. It seems, too, that despite the fact that a rule-out of an anxiety disorder is required to give an ADHD/ADD diagnosis, "professionals" are handing out stimulants like candy, especially to privileged families of historically high-achieving young adults. I have seen that lead to lots more messes that need cleaning up down the road: tolerance, addiction, selling or giving it away, manic episodes, and kids just not believing they have capabilities to be successful without it long after they haven't needed it, *if* they ever did.

The other stressor I see around grades is perfectionism. So many young adults today have forgotten that a B is above average – literally. B's are more often viewed by this age group now as "might as well have failed." They are obviously getting messages from somewhere that it's A's or nothing, and they think about their grades constantly, which is both caused by and causing anxiety. Even if you think "not my kid" because their grades have been mediocre for a while, maybe forever, check in on what their actual capabilities are by getting an assessment. One of the major coping tactics used by young adults who believe it's an A or nothing, is not trying before they can "fail." Yep, if a kid was thought of and/or called "smart" when they were younger, they often perceive that any task that requires *any* amount of effort threatens their view of themselves as smart because smart people don't struggle, right? This tendency to give up without trying is more prevalent in females. There is a fascinating TED Talk by Reshma Saujani about teaching girls bravery over perfection.

Of course, there is nothing wrong with doing one's best and striving for excellence and achievement, but sometimes setting the bar too high can be so overwhelming to a young adult (in fact *any*one) that it causes paralysis. The kid doesn't have a clue where to start, so they don't. In cases like that, the only effective thing may be to lower the bar – perhaps even to below their former or believed capabilities – to a place the student feels confident in their capabilities and then build up from there at a slow but steady pace. There is more to life than grades; however, this treatment strategy often leads to optimal achievement of the student, whatever that is for them. Don't get me wrong, I think most kids oughta be afraid to come home with D's and F's, but a C every once in a while isn't going to keep them out of a good college. And if they do get a lower grade than you (and they) believe they are capable of, start with discussing why and maybe think about getting them assessed before assuming it's "laziness."

Note: I don't believe in laziness as it is widely thought of and used. I believe that what we call "laziness" is a behavior that results from one of two unmanaged emotions. Can you guess which ones? The first is fear (the paralysis that comes with overwhelm, "I don't know where to start, so I won't") and the second is anger (which we'll get into later), which comes out as "F you. I'm not doing that." The "lazy" person may not be able to define which one it is or even that it is emotionally driven, and lazy ends the exploration of that before it even begins.

Social

This one might have been mentioned first because it's debatable which is more important to teens and young adults − grades or friends. There are few things that'll knock a kid down faster and lower into a funk than shit goin' down with friends at school. This probably seems obvious to you, but I have actually been on the phone with a worried dad that said to me, "I mean...it actually seems like [teen] cares more about hanging out with her friend than getting good grades."

Well, duh.

Friends are everything in high school, and they have a huge impact on college life and beyond. Strong positive connections with people are now being linked to life expectancy, optimal cognitive functioning, less illness, and an increase in quality of life. Now, I think there's a lot of back and forth high drama, and they're friends and now they're not, and if you agree with that I strongly suggest you keep that to yourself or your kid'll never again tell you another problem they have with a peer. Remember your validation statements: "Just ignore them" or "Kill 'em with kindness" is *not* a validation statement. Remember, you don't have to agree, you just need to meet them where they are and continue to listen. "That sucks" or "That doesn't sound very kind" will work. You may even attempt a guess at their feelings in a validation statement like, "Seems like you're angry about that," but beware the guess that misses the mark or hits the mark while they're not ready for that truth. It could backfire. Don't push it. Just regroup with something like, "Ok, well…how *do* you feel about it?" No biggie. Back to listening, because along with what seems to you like nonsense and drama, you may pick up some little tidbit that tips you off to some real distress your kid is experiencing. And males – and even those who now identify as male – are socialized to bottle up most negative feelings besides anger and need to be encouraged to talk about their feelings around socializing. Their distress may present differently, like escaping into video games (some with others online), and if you show some genuine interest in the *game* (the thing that is important to them) and you get into open conversation, you may again pick up some clues as to interpersonal conflict that's affecting them negatively. You'd be surprised how much relationship troubles affect males, too.

And every young adult experiences intense sadness when a romantic relationship ends, so by the time that happens, you want to have established some level of open communication because your kid is probably experiencing a heartbreak that is so real and intense for them that that's where other problems they might be having can all culminate into a crisis. Self-harm and break-ups go hand in hand for young people. Cutting may be more prevalent in females and those who identify as female, but self-harm is as common in males. It may not be cutting, but more often presents as fighting, video games, dropping grades, and withdrawal from friends and extra-curricular activities. Even though you may not have considered the romantic relationship as important or healthy (you may even be relieved it's over), you do want to validate them and talk to your kid about how they are experiencing it and what negative emotions they can identify: sadness, regret, anger, hopelessness, etc.

A willingness to actively listen to your kid may reveal to you that they are being bullied at school. As you probably know, bullying is no longer limited to boys beating up other boys and stealing their lunch money. The varied forms and levels of bullying that go on for these kids is alarming. Physical fights do still go on, and are not limited to one gender (or any gender, for that matter). Fighting can be groups or several on one or one on one. The fighting can be driven by many different factors: gender, lack of gender, race, sexual orientation/fluidity, or physical/learning/cognitive differences.

Cyberbullying is the biggest difference in the bullying that goes on with younger generations than our own. The bullying that goes on online actually blows my mind. The psychological distance provided by typing onto a screen has allowed groups of bullies to write heinous things they would otherwise never have the gall to say to that person's face. I think it's a kind of "coward culture" that is hurting lots and lots of kids of all ages. As a parent, the most insidious part is that it all goes on behind closed doors. Parents are often shocked to find out how their kids are using the internet: posting party pics on

Instagram with bottles of booze in plain sight and their kid obviously wasted; Finstagram, which are fake Instagram accounts where (often college) students post more intimate things including, but not limited to, how much they are struggling with suicidal inclinations in kind of an emo-glorification of mental health "diagnoses" and struggles; sending or receiving of dick pics; sending or receiving nude photos (which, if under eighteen, can be considered child pornography); sending or receiving hate speech; sending or receiving a public post instructing another student to "just kill yourself."

Parents, please pay attention: *these are not one-offs*. This is rampant, and I'd be more surprised if your kid did not have one of these happen than if they said they did. But they often don't tell their parents, they tell me. Another set of eyes on your kid will help supplement the attempts you make for more communication with your kid about their friend group.

Non-Majority

There are still cliques of sorts in high school, college, and beyond. The names or types have changed, along with what they consider "cool," but it's only really important to know the haves and the have nots are still in effect. What parents of multiple generations have told their kids of all ages is: *just be yourself*. Yes, I 100 percent agree. I agree that *any* human's lifelong challenge, work, and practice is to learn to take an honest look at themselves, accept their strengths and weaknesses alike, practice liking, loving, and taking good care of themselves through healthy choices and compassion for mistakes, and expand and grow. Yes. 100 percent.

The problem comes with the reality that we are all unique in who we are – which, ironically, makes us all alike. But that's not really how the world works, is it? There are groups of people of all ages who are not part of majority groups. And when you're not part of a majority group, you have challenges the majority doesn't have – now times a thousand if you're still developing as a human aged eleven to twenty-six, let's say.

Your female kid has to deal with the negative feelings she experiences due to sexism. She may experience fear of rape and sexual assault every day, and has likely been sexually assaulted at school multiple times. She may be called on less in the classroom and feel frustrated by that. She probably doesn't like her body and has engaged in disordered eating on multiple occasions. And yes, she most likely has at least tried cutting to cope with all these stressors.

Your kid may be hiding from you that they're queer. Have you ever suspected your kid might be gay? Would you be ok with that? They may not identify with assignments given at their birth, like their sex, gender, or name. They have to deal with the stress of school and probably fear of homophobic threats – physical, verbal, and on the internet. Your kid may be very, very isolated, which is always a red flag, and makes them feel lonely, and maybe self-loathing. They may be cutting. Or they may think about suicide. Or they may wonder if you or others will still love them if they "Just Be Themselves."

If your kid is a person of color (POC) and you are a person of color, you already know that institutional racism is a stressor that white people will never experience. Does your kid talk to you about hate speech they experience at school or online? Your kid may be toughing it out alone and need to talk. Would you be ok sending them to therapy? How about with a white therapist? (More about this later, but you already know....whoa...choose wisely.)

And if you were born in another country and your kid was born here, what differences are you prepared to tolerate in them that don't mean to you you're "losing them?" Your kid may feel anxiety and shame about being between cultural groups and not being "_____ enough." Are you ok with your kid having friends of another race?

Your kid with physical differences or cognitive/developmental differences is probably struggling with bullying and degradation at school, and you probably actively worry about that. What you may not know is that your teen or young adult thinks about sex, too. How do you talk to them about their sexuality? Has a caregiver or teacher suggested independent living? Are there potential benefits to your kid's growth to living on their own, even though your heart rate just skyrocketed reading that?

And, of course, there are so many ways these kids and stressors intersect − if you are straight and white, please think about that for a minute. If you are male and you were born here, please think about that for a minute. There are many other stressors specific to varying circumstances: chronic illness, adoption, parents of different race or cultures, to name a few. A lot of times the more of these non-majority boxes you tick, the more the compounded anxiety, depression, and anger.

Anger

I have found in my fifteen years of treating people, specifically young people who self-harm, that the number one factor that unifies all the ways they hurt themselves and all the different stress factors among all the unique kids is ineffective management of their experience of anger. You may find this surprising since, so far throughout this book, I've been referring to anxiety and depression as the emotions leading to cutting. Let me get into it here.

Anxiety is almost always a factor when someone is cutting themselves. I have found that few things spike anxiety like stuffed anger. I have had participants I work with come in with chronic self-harm behaviors and cutting, *and* frequent and debilitating panic attacks. They may have been cutting on and off for a while, maybe they haven't cut themselves in years, or maybe they still cut themselves weekly, but what brings them through my door for the first time are the panic attacks. They're having them at school, work, home. They're fearing one coming on, even when they're not having them. We've tracked the timing, the situation(s), the patterns of onset of the panic attack, and after years of seeing this, we almost always uncover buried rage, like, years-long stuffed anger. They've been so afraid of the anger they've chronically avoided dealing with it and now it inevitably erupts from inside 'em. They even resist my initial theory that it may be related to anger.

Mind you, they're *desperate* to stop having panic attacks. They literally think they will die during a panic attack, come in begging for help, yet immediately dismiss the idea that anger may play a role. They don't always even know they're doing that- it's just so ingrained in them, for one old reason or another, to deny their experience of anger. I'm telling you, time and time again we do some really tough anger work, which requires a lot of *unlearning* and a shit-ton of courage on their part, and many never have another panic attack again. And some do when they stuff their anger again. Then they understand that there is some choice and control in their management of both anger *and* anxiety. So, with cutting (even without panic attacks) there is a relationship between anxiety and anger and engaging in self-harming behaviors. We see the unhealthy behaviors decrease as the new healthy tools are understood, taught, and practiced.

Depression can often work the same way with kids (or just people) that cut. I think of anxiety and depression as basically two sides of the same coin, and there is so much attention paid by MDs in treating depression that I think very often the anxiety that almost always fuels, or is a factor in depression, is missed. I talk about this with my participants and let them know there is, indeed, a difference between clinical depression and what I call "anxiety burnout."

It's worth noting that anxiety is an emotion under the umbrella of fear. But depression is not an emotional experience, it's a diagnosis: a pathological condition. Most people use the word depression interchangeably with "sadness" which is mostly a naturally occurring emotional experience. People say, "I was feeling a little depressed today," until I make this point and they tweak the language. People have been so conditioned to look at depression as common and normal instead of a treatable diagnosis that they forget that they sometimes feel sad… and that's ok.

Anxiety burnout is the paralysis that comes from overwhelm. Remember before when I said I don't believe in laziness? That laziness is either the result of strong feelings of fear or anger? Well, if someone's in bed all the time, we automatically think they might be depressed, right? But, what I see just as often is more of a "hiding" from the world. The ol' "I don't know where to start so I won't," which many people rationalize into "I can't" or "There's no point anyway," so it gets mistaken for depression instead of anxiety. Also, have you ever heard the saying "depression is anger turned inward"? Turns out there's some truth to that and again, in the case of someone being "lazy" and staying in bed all the time. It may be overwhelm but it could also be the digging the heels in of anger: "Fuck you. I'm not doing that" or "Life is stupid and a waste" or "Everything I do amounts to nothing."

Again, this looks like what we call depression, and it may well be! But when I've done the anger work with folx that cut and maybe also stay in bed or have panic attacks or many other symptoms and problems, we find so much there. So, why are people so afraid of anger? It's just an emotion like any other emotion. Anger is the emotion that alerts us that our boundaries are being crossed or violated, so it's so important to learn how to identify when we feel anger. Anger can help us stay emotionally and even physically safe. I think people worry feeling and naming anger will lead to them blowing up uncontrollably and looking like an asshole. Funny thing is, the complete opposite is true. Naming anger validates our emotional experience and gives us the chance to learn tools for effectively managing anger and *choosing* how we want to handle our anger. It's the lack of awareness of anger and denial of its existence that lead to outbursts and tantrums and choices that bite us in the ass later and cause shame. Without the anger work, I seriously have no idea how anyone who cuts themselves stops. I haven't seen that ever happen. Anger work does take a bit, though. It's a process you really don't want to rush. Long gone are the days where psychologists thought family therapy with padded bats was a healthy move. The general thought these days is that pushing someone into intense bursts of anger on purpose is harmful and often leads to more uncontrolled anger.

So, we don't poke the bear in my office. We take it at a pace that is uncomfortable and challenging, yet tolerable...sometimes even slower than that. In Chapter 8 we'll get you some tools for handling that ride, but first let's tackle this question of to medicate or not to medicate in Chapter 7.

CHAPTER 7
MEDS ARE NOT AUTOMATIC

First off, I am a psychologist not a psychiatrist, so I legally cannot make recommendations regarding medication. I can only tell you what I've seen and my opinion as a non-MD.

The first suggestion most other clinicians – both psychologists and psychiatrists – are going to make to you if your kid is cutting is meds. Psychotropic medication is an option for depression and anxiety, and that *may* be what your kid ends up needing and it *may* help your kid. The danger, in my opinion, is the trend to over-pathologize teens and young adults, particularly if they're female, a person of color, or trans- to over-medicalize cutting and other self-harm behaviors, and to over-medicate the people that engage in cutting.

Don't get me wrong, meds do help many people and many people would suffer greatly without 'em. I take issue with the amount of meds freely given to people whose brains and bodies are still growing. The truth is we really don't know what that does to a person's brain. The brain is still largely unknown and the vast majority of psychiatrists grossly underplay what a crapshoot meds are. I also don't think meds "cure" every, or even many, psychological issue that teens are grappling with. I had a teen come in on eight different psych meds – *eight* – and she was still really off the rails behaviorally and she was cutting. The psychiatrist just kept adding another medication every time she'd act out. Now, tell me, what medication do you think is best for walking in and seeing your mother mid-suicide attempt? A benzo for anxiety? An antidepressant? Something for sleep? (To be fair, the therapist she was seeing told her to do "therapeutic hand gestures," which is worse than a meds crapshoot, in my opinion.)

Psychiatrists just keep adding medications and most are very reluctant to take someone *off* because of liability issues. Bluntly, if they titrate down the meds and the kid suicides, the psychiatrists fear litigation. I wish there was something they feared enough to be that cautious *before* putting the kid on meds. So just consider that part before automatically medicating your kids. I have worked with a couple of psychiatrists that will work with the kids I see and have safely gotten them off *all* their meds, even when they started on anything from three to eight different daily ones. Very few MDs will do that, and even fewer tell parents no when they bring their kids in for a first appointment and are pissed they paid for it and left "empty-handed." I, clinically and personally, don't think such things ought to be evaluated like a business transaction...it's a kid's brain we're talking about for fuck's sake. You can draw your own conclusions, but having the facts makes for an educated decision and you do have alternatives to meds.

In my work with teens and young adults, the vast majority who came in miserable, cutting, and on meds stopped cutting within a couple of months – not years – got off most or all their meds, and are now doing the work confidently and joyfully with me or on their own.

Ok, so when you discover your kid is cutting themselves here is a pretty straight-forward protocol of questions you need to ask and get answers for:

Hospitalization: Does Your Kid Need to Go to the Hospital for Cutting?

Questions: Well, do they need stitches? Did they cut themselves, pass out, and hit their head? Are they telling you they want to die?

My Answer: If you are unsure about any of these questions, it's probably a good idea to get your kid assessed by admit at the ER. If all are no's, you probably don't have to go, but if you're still unsure you absolutely can.

Potential Downside: The downside is that it's on your kid's permanent medical record and if they admit your kid, it may be involuntary. Obviously, if any of the above questions are a yes, you gotta go to the emergency room anyway and it's worth it. It's if they are no's that you may be on the fence. Another *potential* downside is that your kid will most likely come out of the hospital on meds... possibly over-medicated.

Potential Upside: If your kid is suicidal, they will be safe from hurting themselves in the hospital. If they really need to be there, it's containing and they go to programs, maybe even some version of DBT, and they might be offered a place in a partial hospitalization program (PHP) or other outpatient services. If they don't need to be there, the hospital can be a pretty scary and awful experience and if they think they will be sent there every time they cut themselves, they may stop cutting themselves. Strategic consequences *do* often work.

Wilderness Training Programs: Does Your Kid Need to Be Sent into a Wilderness Program?

(i.e., picked up from your house and taken to a therapeutic program that's like inpatient in that they cannot leave, but in nature. They are usually at least several months long.)

Questions: Are things getting outta hand at home? Is your kid who's cutting themselves disrupting the entire family unit? Is the cutting behavior chronic? Is your kid also running away? Has your kid become unruly and no longer regards you with respect or authority?

My Answer: Well, you get that if these are all yes's it's probably time. If you keep them at home it means most of your answers are no's and your kid has professional help and they are progressing.

Potential Downside: *You must research.* Google it, ask a professional, or hire a consultant. It's my general understanding that Wilderness Programs have largely cleaned up their acts and the those with reports of abuse have been shut down. These programs are very expensive and often the step-down is therapeutic boarding school which is also very expensive. Also, if your kid has to be taken at night because of flight-risk, they may have problems sleeping in the future.

Potential Upside: The only Wilderness program I can professionally vouch for is Open Sky in Durango, Colorado. I have been on site in the woods, observed programmatic activities, and spent time with administration. They use DBT, which I obviously think is effective, and observed a level of understanding of its practice that I have only ever seen in my office – and from Dr. Lenihan herself. They are one of the few programs which require parent participation, which I think is bold and necessary.

Should Your Kid See a General Practitioner (GP) or Naturopath?

Questions: Is something physiological going on that's causing the cutting?

My Answer: From what I've seen, not often. But, I do have a colleague who says her depression went away when she removed gluten from her diet, so let's just make sure.

Potential Downside: The MD makes some dismissive comment about cutting that reveals a lack of understanding or caring or even really listening to, looking at, or believing your kid and wants to put them on meds without a talk therapy referral…my pet-peeve.

Potential Upside: Get the data! Insist the MD (PA, NP, or Naturopath) order full blood work, a urine (and stool) test, and test for food allergies. You're here for rule-outs, for psychotropic medication get assessed by a specialist: a psychiatrist.

Mental Health: Does My Kid Need Psychotherapy/ Talk Therapy or Meds?

Questions: Are they cutting themselves but somewhat still functional, or not?

My Answer: I absolutely do not agree with putting a teen or young adult on brain chemical-altering drugs without talk therapy. Period. A decent psychiatrist will agree with that, too. Meds are for helping a person level out to a point where talk therapy has a chance to be effective. Please do not try to use a psychiatrist for anything but medication management. They think they can do talk therapy. They can't. MDs don't listen. Active, empathic listening is integral to talk therapy's efficacy, and if your kid is cutting, they do need to talk to a professional who understands the complicated psychology around self-harm behaviors (more in Chapter 9).

Potential Downside: You get a useless narcissist who doesn't help and costs you a shitload of money. Your kid may get misdiagnosed with the latest trendy diagnosis (and possibly get sent for unnecessary meds), get worse, and now doesn't trust talk therapy.

Potential Upside: You find the right fit for your kid for talk therapy and don't need to put them on meds and not only do they stop cutting themselves, they learn tools for coping that increase instead of decrease their sense of confidence and self-esteem, and they grow into a healthy adult that loves and respects themselves. Not hyperbole. I've seen evidence many times.

It's tough to navigate the field of mental health, doctors, programs, and pills...not to mention the broken system of insurance, which is even worse regarding mental health. The good news is when you find a talk therapy professional that's a match for your kid, you can see progress sooner than you might have guessed. I'll maximize your chances of that very thing in Chapter 9, but if the professional and your kid are doing productive work, that means it's going to get bumpy. That's what we'll address next in Chapter 8.

CHAPTER 8
WORSE BEFORE BETTER

The veteran clinicians I was in private practice with for so many years had a saying: "Change is Bad." Everyone would laugh at the paradox. I slowly began to realize, as I made the transition from the first practicum student they'd accepted, to the eager, bright-eyed pre-doc intern, to the admiring post-doc, to the reverent licensed staff member, to the driven staff and board member, that they weren't fully joking. As creator of the DBT program, I wasn't a proponent of black and white languaging like "good/bad," "right/wrong," "worthwhile/worthless," but I thought that reductive wording was part of the joke.

Nope.

I announced, back when I was made staff, that I was going to push for real change, and when it fell on deaf-ears long enough for me to take my edict to the board, I realized that this group, whose core members had done things a certain way since before I was born, really did practice a "change is bad" way of life. So I, in heart-break, needed to move on – into a place I didn't know:

not just private practice, but a *way* of practicing that I now knew was far, far from the norm, even for supposedly one of the most open and progressive towns in the country. And it's one of the most painful and beneficial experiences of my adult life.

I will say this...change is *hard*. Not all the time, but often. The sudden stuff, the events that rock us to our core and require true acts of bravery in order to come through 'em, is the most transformative. We know we're a better version of ourselves for having had the courage to face it, instead of hide. One of my favorite bands, the Trashcan Sinatras, have this one song with the lyrics I often share with my participants: "Out of harm's way, where the traps all lay..." They're Scottish, so you can easily miss it, and I never could quite get to a confident place with the whole lay/lie-thing – despite all the Catholic schooling of proper grammar. But I often think of that line in times of strife and try to ride that painful wave 'til calmer and clearer waters arrive.

This is what I ask of you now. Your kid is cutting. You're developing a plan. The most efficient plan with the deepest and most long-term benefits deems that things get worse before they get better. I'll tell you what I tell almost every person I've ever worked with: "I'm sorry about that. That's the reality of it. If I could have found an easier way through, I would have found it by now."

So, strap in. It's gonna get bumpy.

First, as I said earlier, with cutting there is inevitably anger work that needs to get done. It's not pretty for *anybody*. And when your kid is paraphrasing some point I made with them in our work together and using it against you in a heated conflict, you gotta hang in there and trust that they will get through. You will all get through it. In sessions, I liken the anger work to the *Shawshank Redemption*. Have you seen that movie? Well, basically, Andy DuFresne spends years planning how to escape from prison (he's innocent, by the way) and the actual night comes when he has his chance. He has to open up a pipe of raw human sewage, climb *into* said sewage pipe, *crawl* some ungodly distance (I think they measure it in football fields in the movie), even vomiting as he goes, until he gets to the stream at the end of the pipe. It's raining, and the shot looks down on him as he raises his arms to the thunder and lightning in an epic gesture of freedom. Yeah, *you* are Andy DuFresne in this scenario. The anger work that your kid has to go through puts your whole family in the shit tunnel. When you keep going, even if you *will* get through it. And you will be free.

The conflicts that your kid will instigate with you as they're figuring out how to navigate their anger will not be pretty. If they were a chronic stuffer before, chances are they'll *also* overshoot the acknowledging their anger part. The pendulum tends to swing wide before balancing out, ya know what I'm sayin'? Just know, that I am *also* in the third ring of Dante's inferno – hell, that is – with your kid. I've already built a "safe space" and connection with them to say whatever's authentically going on with them, and this is the time I'm *almost* regretting how "safe" they feel to express themselves. They're being little assholes to me, too, y'know. And I *engage* in the horn-lock with them. I make sure I win- for *them*, so they can continue to experience the safety of knowing where the lines are and what *consequences* they will expect if they choose to cross that line. (We will go heavily into consequences in Chapter 10). You will also need to engage in the horn-lock with them, and for their sake you must "win." I'll get into some tips on effective communication, but first let's get into what *not* to do during this process, shall we?

Your communication with your kid was already probably somewhat limited because of their age and their tendency to hide unhealthy behaviors like cutting. I earnestly ask that you assume a *"please"* preceding the following bullet points:

- *Do not* guilt-trip. Just don't do it. They already are mired in shame about their self-harm and whatever else they think they're fucking up. Don't bring up how you used to get along so well, or they used to tell you things, or they used to be happy. It doesn't work anyway, and can actually make them feel worse and interact with you *less*.

- *Do not* use phrases that refer to their cutting as "just to get attention," because you know what? You're right. Your kid needs some attention paid to the distress they are experiencing because they don't have the tools and emotional intelligence and maturity to deal with it themselves. Don't kick 'em while they're down, Dude.

- *Do not* tell your kid they are "being dramatic." Your kid obviously perceives they are being ignored in some way, so they thought they needed to "amp up" whatever behavior(s) would get them the airtime they believe they need. They did that because they think their feelings are not valid. Don't further invalidate their feelings of distress by then minimizing their pain.

- *Do not* refer to your kid as "too sensitive," especially reactively to something you just said to them that they perceived as hurtful. First of all, it is *my* job to build up their ego-strength, resilience, and ability to shake things off. You're too close to them to do that job. Your kid, no matter how old they get, will always desire your approval. Your words are more powerful to them than any other person they will ever meet in their lives...no exaggeration. They supremely care what you think of them. Second, what I'd like to know is when the hell did sensitive get twisted into something negative? Is sensitivity too feminine a trait and so we need to systematically denigrate that trait to ensure the patriarchy stays intact? Asking for a friend. The one thing I will tell you if your kid cuts, they feel big. They have a huge heart, and their emotions are an important part of how they live their lives. Lucky, actually. You heard me right. Yes, of course all that intensity of emotion is hurting them (and they're currently hurting *themselves* because of it), but once they learn the tools to identify, manage, and *direct* all those emotions, they are capable of some incredible things. They will be our future's artists, humanitarians, statespeople, leaders...do-gooders, basically. I call it the "Bunnies & Rainbows Team." Those of us who believe we're on the earth to develop our unique talents to later use in service to humanity. That's probably your kid. So let's get 'em on that track. Get all those strong emotions directed into a positive endeavor. And that *requires* a special "sensitivity," so let's not shame them for their superpower, eh?

Now the Do's:

- *Please do* thank the kid for being your kid.

- *Do* validate *all* of the feelings they are brave and open enough to express to you. Remember: the feelings, the *emotions* are all valid. The thoughts generated from the emotions are *not* necessarily valid. Fear is a liar. It tricks us into all kinds of nutty thoughts that are not necessarily true, and if we believe those thoughts generated by fear and worry, we may *act* from that with impulsive *behaviors*, which we don't validate either. (Rick Carson does a great job explaining this in his book *Taming Your Gremlin*.)

- When your kid presents a problem they're having (which is rare and brave already), what do we do? We *validate* them *before* problem solving, as discussed in Chapter 4. It might look something like this: kid expresses complaint about school, and you might say, "That sounds hard. Can I help, or do you just wanna vent?" And if it's the latter, just listen without offering advice.

- *Do* use effective ways of communicating with your kid. They are not a child anymore. Validation, but also try this DBT exercise:

- https://docs.wixstatic.com/ugd/87024e_ d81580ee4dc74ec994bebfbeeb5c20d6.pdf write it out, practice out loud. It works with bosses and spouses, too. You're welcome!

- *Do* go get some parent coaching. Co-parent from a shared model that you learned from an experienced professional.

- *Do* go out for dinner afterward...you deserve a reward for weathering all this hard work!

And even more crucial than you finding the right parenting coach, is finding just the right professional to help your kid out of the muck. The next chapter deals with that.

CHAPTER 9
GET THE RIGHT FIT

When you discover your kid is cutting, I cannot overstate the importance of these two things:

1. Get your kid's ass in therapy *right now*! That means, like, yesterday. Ya dig? This cutting behavior has gone on awhile, regardless of what your kid has told you. And before your kid was actually engaging in self-harm behavior, they were thinking about it for a while before *that*. Your kid has been struggling for a long time before your discovery of their cutting. Whatever they are distressed about may have been or may still *be* unknown to *them*. It's going to take a professional – someone trained in sifting through these layers of emotions – to help your kid navigate their way outta this bloody mess.

2. Get your kid hooked up with a psychologist that has a specialty in teens and young adults and seems "real." Yeah, you can search online parents' networks, and definitely peruse their own

website, but make sure you speak to them live – on the phone, Zoom, in person…it doesn't matter, just so it's in real time. Listen for anything that appears somewhat "off-script" and authentic – if they're slightly abrupt – possibly all the better (but I'm biased).

So how do you achieve these two important goals?

- You shop. Yep, you are the consumer. So shop around. Make a bunch of appointments with researched clinicians, and preferably word-of-mouth referrals. I tell all parents and kids during the first appointment, "If you and I don't jive, keep shopping!" Hint: some of the best ones don't take insurance and you often get what you pay for, but not always. There is a sea of mediocrity out there, and it's *all* expensive.

- There is no debate on whether the kid is going to therapy. They *are* going – it's a non-negotiable – find the leverage. You can take away privileges and/or enforce consequences if they continue to fight you. More on how in Chapter 10. I've had kids physically dragged to their first meeting with me, or lied to that they're going to get ice cream. Real nice set-up for our relationship based on trust, right? But I make it work. I once met such a pissed off teen that they were so slumped down in the chair they were damn near horizontal. I stuck my hand out to shake theirs as an intro. One finger of one hand that gripped the arm rest was raised.

I shook it. We went across the street to my office, and, gracefully as ever, I tripped going up the stairs. I heard a gasp and an immediate, "Are you ok?" in earnest from the kid. The walls were down. True colors were shown. Tough to put them back up after that. I figure, better they're there and pissed off than not there at all. They *do not* get a reward for going, though. Therapy is still a privilege, and bribery is enabling. You are the boss.

- You can leave it up to your teen or young adult to choose the psychologist, but there is no choice in going to *someone*. And once they choose, they can't request to go back to "shopping" once the hard work begins. Remember, a couple of weeks or months in, if the professional is challenging your kid, they may want to flee to avoid conflict with the clinician. Sometimes kids even have an impulse to quit because of conflict. Fine, if they are going to quit, at least make them go do it in person. That's usually when the kid and I bust through to something important and they pretty much never think seriously of quitting again.

- They are then in charge of and responsible for scheduling if aged fourteen and over, in my opinion, because their therapy is their responsibility.

- If they skip, *they* pay the no-show fee and call the clinician themselves to apologize and reschedule. They can work it off at home – with cleaning, filing, yard work – whatever you need done (more in Chapter 10).

- Other than skipping and working off the fee, *do not* talk to your kid about how much therapy costs. This goes with my earlier point of No Guilt Tripping. Since your kid is cutting themselves, believe me, they already think they are unworthy of the cost of therapy. Please, *please* do not burden them with the concept of adult financial responsibilities. They cannot handle it. They already feel guilty and anxious and think they're a burden to you.

- Although it's perfectly natural to feel some amount of jealousy toward your kid's relationship with their clinician, since they may be telling me things you wish they'd tell you, *do not* act out those feelings. Parents implore me to work with their kids to help them stop cutting, only to let jealousy creep in a month or two later with a not-so-subtle competitive comment to their kid. Don't be that parent. I don't give a shit what you think of me, personally, but if your kid is in a therapeutic relationship with me and chest-deep in the scary emotional work, they depend on me for their emotional guidance and health. One petty comment can cause an inner conflict for your kid where they feel torn and guilty and anxious about trusting me, like it's some kind of betrayal of you. That can be so destructive, that if you fully understood it, you would never even dream of doing that to your adult child. Stick with the plan and model dignified and brave behavior while your kid heals.

While the clinician does the psychological work with your kid, you can empower yourself and get the whole family unified in positive and healthy action with a well thought out plan. I'll teach you how in Chapter 10.

CHAPTER 10
BUILD THE PLAN

Ok, so you have the professional in place to start the ball rollin' on your kid's recovery. Now we can get on to your job. Just like I teach the participants I work with the tools for building their confidence, courage, and a joyful life, so, too, will I help you build your toolbox for helping your kid not only stop cutting, but continue to progress into adulthood with confidence, a solid set of values to guide them, self-respect, and joy. So let's get to the plan!

Expectations

The cornerstone of the plan is that you get *very clear* about your expectations of your kid as a member of your household. We need to define our objectives here. What are their jobs/chores around the house? What do you expect their grades to be? Do they have a job outside of the house? What are their privileges? What happens if they don't meet expectations? How do you support the success of this plan as a parent or parents?

Contracts

All these and more questions need to be answered and they need to be written down. You write up a contract and include each section of this chapter: expectations, privileges, consequences…all the specifics. Then you sit down, with your kid. You read over all the points in the contract aloud. You make sure your kid understands each point – mind you, they need not *agree* with the points. *You* have already decided and it's not up for debate. Get verbal confirmation from them that they understand (a salty head-nod will do). Once you get through the entire contract, parent or parents *and* kid will sign and date the contract and then it will be kept on the fridge in full view so it can be referenced in any argument where "I didn't know" or "You never said that" gets thrown around. It also holds you to the original boundaries you put in place when you're feeling some guilt or worry about enforcing consequences or "droppin' the hammer," as I call it. The idea is that we want to reduce the amount of mood-dependent decision making that goes on around these issues. Emotions fly around with parents and teens/young adults, es*pecially* when cutting is happening. That drives emotional intensity *way* up. So we want to develop the contract when you're calm, collected, logical, and clear on your family's core values. So that you have a tool to ground you back down when the emotional heat gets turned up…and it will.

Grades

Assuming your kid is in high school, college, or grad school (even if your grad student doesn't live in your houschold, if you financially support them, you have a right to expectations around grades) what is reasonable to expect from your kid's grades? I assume since your kid is cutting that it's likely their grades have been slipping, if not tanking. If they haven't, this section may not take much time – but still do it in case slipping happens later.

We base these grades expectations on their average academic history, any data you've collected from testing (neuropsych, academic, etc.), and a small percentage on what you believe they are capable of getting. What expectation is *not* based on is what you *wish* your kid's grades were. Straight A's are not within everyone's reach, and that's ok! Frankly, most of the kids I see that get straight A's have some major perfectionistic tendencies, *tons* of anxiety issues, and don't have much of a clue how to let their hair down and have fun. You'd think, as a parent, that that would be a dream come true, but believe me... it isn't for the kid (and the adult they become). Yes, we want them to work hard and do their best. Of course we do. We just want some well-roundedness in there, too, and self-esteem intact, please. And will you name letter grades, or a general grade point average? Yes, it needs to be that specific. And it needs to be class by class and therefore changed each semester, trimester, or quarter.

I do straight B's with participants, but you need not agree with that. I like straight B's because if that seems too low for the kid, then great! They should have no trouble meeting it and getting the self-esteem points for accomplishing a goal they committed to. That's when we usually can see if they still stress themselves out even with that relatively low expectation. I think the kids that work hard and have consistent and useful study habits don't also need to freak out, but they often do anyway. So we work on trusting in themselves, not behaving like a lemming or a martyr – there's no virtue in being like everybody else or in unnecessary suffering. Be grateful for your brain and work ethic and chill the fuck out. That's one path.

If the straight B's are higher than the kid has been getting, but it's around what they used to get before they were cutting and in crisis, then we're just working on how to get the grades back up. What are the practical tweaks we need to make in your kid's day to day that will lead to accomplishing B's and where are those choice points where fear tricks them into picking the unhealthy choice? We systematically figure that out and change in baby steps. That's the other path.

The last path is the one where the kid never really got straight B's at their healthiest – and that's ok, too. Perhaps there are some learning differences and testing could help, and/or maybe academia just isn't their thing. When that's the case we do what it takes to graduate with dignity – cooperatively setting goals for grades that make sense- and we look at trades and other career options that don't require more school and bring in an income sustainable for where and how they want to live.

You already have an idea of where your kid falls, but talk to them about it. What do they want to do? How do they want to live? They may not know, but it's not a bad idea to begin to think about that; not in a pressured way, just a conversation. And I'm always checking on grades with my participants anyway, because it tells me a lot about their psychological well-being; where their strengths are and what needs tweaking. If your kid's grades *have* tanked recently, they're going to need some extra support for a while. If you can afford a tutor, just spare yourself the nightly power-struggle and headache and hire one. Tutors are really great for academic help, but especially to enforce accountability, organization, and time management. You will not regret it. If a tutor is not in your budget, is there free help at school? Many schools have free after-school services, or peer-run check-in help. If your kid is away at college, they can speak to their advisor about where to get help and check the student assistance center. There are lots of options, the point is don't *not* get them support. If your kid lives at home, I strongly suggest nightly homework check-ins and that you put that in the contract. It's a pain in the ass for you and for them, but until they can demonstrate that they don't need it, this is how it's got to be. Chin up – it's temporary.

Chores

No matter what your income and means, your kid *must* have regular duties that they are responsible for as a contributing member of your household. Period. If you have can afford to hire someone to come in and clean, that's great – they are not to do the kid's chores for them, even if they do a better job than your kid does. Example: their bedroom. The hired cleaner can do the floors in the kid's room, but only if they can *see* a floor. Maybe the kid's nightly job is to clear the dinner table and fill the dishwasher – great. They are to do that without a reminder and without pissin' and moanin'. How? We'll get into that in the privileges & consequences section. But for now, just figure out what your expectations are and put them in the contract. We'll get to how to enforce it later. If you're considering outsourcing a project around the house, think about whether or not to put that on your kid's chore list, and I'd keep a running chore list on the fridge next to the contract (or on a bulletin board or white board or however your family does it).

If, and it *is* an "if," you choose to bring in an allowance to this chore situation, that has to be specifically outlined in the contract. How much, for what, in what amount of time, how much is taken away if something isn't finished in the allotted time…all of it. You *also* have to be prepared to not give it to them if they don't complete their commitments. Might I suggest first implementing the basic contract, and once that's smoothly rollin' for a month or so, come back to the allowance debate. It could muddy the waters if brought in right away. I prefer it being brought in later because it lands as more of a "bonus" for all the hard work they've been accomplishing. Y'dig?

Part-Time Work

All I really have to say about a job outside of the house is that it's generally a good idea for them to get a job outside the house. The more it sucks, the better because nothing highlights the importance of education like makin' sandwiches or cleanin' toilets. (And no, I'm not being insensitive to blue-collar workers. I did both the entirety of college and I'm not even going mention the landfill I worked at, so don't even.) They think *you're* a tyrant, wait 'til they hear how the assistant manager talks to 'em, and they can't pop-off to *her*. Yeah, it's character building all right. It also takes care of the whole allowance debate because they earn their own going-out money and that's better for them anyway. Here's the *one* thing I will caution about the part-time job outside the house:

The grades must come first. If they are in school, that *is* their job. If your family is in dire times and you need any money any member can bring in, that is, of course, another story. Other than that kind of scenario, a part-time job is a privilege...and privileges are *earned*.

Privileges

Yep, that's right. It seems to be the thing, these days, that privileges are automatic instead of earned. That's about to change. There's a new sheriff in town. If your family has been thrown into a crisis because of cutting and the behaviors that often come with cutting, things need to change. And if there are other kids in the house, of any age, they can follow the plan, too. And it's not the "fault" of the kid who's cutting, it's something that you've decided would be better for the whole family and you "wish you'd put the plan in place long time ago" or whatever just gets them on board. You are the parent(s). *You* make the rules. And if you want to change the rules for the betterment of the family, well by God, you're gonna *do* that. You feel me?

Privileges that, in my book, are *not* automatic:

- Phone (yes, you read that right...*phone)*
- Car
- Laptop (even if it's for school)
- Spending money
- Going out with friends
- Internet – *yes* (it's not that hard to separate school stuff from leisure stuff)

So this is by no means is a complete list. You will make that. And you don't need to agree with my list, you base it on your own family's values. I just wanted to offer you some support in thinking that your kid(s) are not *entitled* to any of these things and *you* bought them so *you* own them. They will disagree, but who gives a rat's arse about *that?* And who's been teaching them that, by the way? You want your kid(s) to act respectfully? Know the value of money? Ask politely and be grateful? Learn time management? Not tantrum as adults when everything doesn't go their way? Of course you do! So get really, *really* clear on what your family considers or *now* considers a privilege. And privileges are earned and can, therefore, be taken away.

Consequences

So, I guess the word "punishment" is out of fashion, and I get it – language does matter. And it's probably progressive that knockin' your kid into next week for mouthing off at the grocery store is out of fashion, too. Time marches on. There is a percentage of the grocery store scenario that I do agree with. And before you lose your shit, I am a survivor of childhood physical and psychological abuse. I am also a practitioner of dialectics – the Venn diagram? And I think that life is *not* as simple as black and white, but is, in fact, gray. I don't believe in child abuse; of course not. But I am not 100 percent against spankings, either- when they are not delivered in anger or meant to degrade or strip dignity.

For our purposes and the purposes of your family's plan, consequences simply means the taking away of privileges. So for a consequence to work, you have to take away a thing your kid cares about – maybe the most. So, if they've been shut down lately, which I see a lot with kids in the throes of cutting, telling them they can't hang out with their friends tonight or they cannot participate in their extra-curricular activity until a chore is done may not work. They might be like, "fine" and not finish the chore and happily take that consequence.

But, if they're blowing off their studies and friends are everything, and you say no internet until your homework is finished, they may think they can be on the computer pretending to do homework, but really they're DMing their friends. That's an easy one. You ask them how long they think their homework will take (let's say two hours), then inform them that you'll be back to check it (and it better match up with their teacher's online program that lists their assignments and when they're due) and then they can be on with their friends for an hour (or whatever timeframe you deem reasonable) after that. You must come in at the agreed upon time and check like you said you would. No consequence is worth a damn without diligent follow-through, which is also why you never want to threaten a kid with a consequence you have no intention of following through on – that's a very quick way to lose credibility with a teen/young adult. So, you go back and see if the homework is done, and if it matches what is due tomorrow and then they get an hour online for pleasure or they don't. By the way, no phone or computer can *ever* be left in the kid's room at night. They turn their phone in to you each night and get it back in the morning. Young people *never* turn off their phones at night because *FOMO!* (Fear of missing out) I'm not kidding. They will be even more sleep-deprived than they already are, and that makes for a cranky kid and a slow recovery. I also suggest getting a padlock small enough to go through the hole in an outlet plug so they are not on a computer all night (laptops, like phones obviously are not left in their room at night). The tiny padlock prevents them from even plugging in a desktop.

The quickest, easiest, and maybe most effective consequence is taking the kid's phone. Whatever chore they haven't done, or whatever violation of curfew or other expectation that's been violated, their wish to have their phone back is powerful enough to make them do damn near anything. I'm sure you already know this, but I suspect you *under*use this as a consequence. Why? What I hear a lot is, "Well, I want to be able to reach them when they're out," as though we've never lived in a world without cell phones. Ok, well maybe they don't *go* out then. *Or*, you keep an old flip-phone on your plan for just such an occasion. You can still buy flip-phones, by the way, and they're cheap. I cannot tell you what an effective consequence that is; it's gold.

Manual Labor as a Consequence

You can ask any of my past or present participants...I am a *huge fan!* You got some leaves out in the yard? The garage need cleaning? Hedges need clipping? Lawn needs mowing? Whatever. The more mundane, the better. I have even encouraged parents to have the kid go out and dig a certain size hole, wait 'til they come in and say they're finished, and then say, "Now go fill it up." Why? Because it's the suckiest thing I could think of at the time. The sheer futility of it makes it a winner. Plus it's exercise. The majority of young people do not get enough physical exercise, and they need it – we all do. Plus, activity that raises the heart rate, even moderately, for a sustained twenty minutes is a mood stabilizer. It mellows out anxiety and lifts/prevents depression. Manual labor is all-around good for 'em. That's a big part of what makes a good wilderness program so effective. See, even my consequences are made of love!

Grounding

My kind of grounding, as you may have guessed, is hardcore. Everything goes. All privileges are suspended until...that's the thing. I think the most important thing about grounding a kid, however you choose to do it, is defining beforehand (ideally in the contract) how long it's going to be. Then you don't flake, they don't beg, and most importantly, there's no shame. You don't say "when things improve." What things? Improve to what? That's way too vague, and it doesn't put the kid in charge of doing their time with their dignity intact. I don't see the psychological benefit your kid gets from you just holding being grounded over their head to get them to do things. No. *Be clear*. What's gone, how long, what kinda time will get tacked on for wheedling/new screw-ups, etc. Every last detail. Clarity is key. It creates a sense of psychological safety for kids to know what's coming if they choose to break the rules. Breaking the rules is part of adolescence – hell, it's part of life. And you want them to know that if when they make that choice they must be prepared to accept the consequences. I call it "learning to eat your shit sandwich with dignity" and I guess that's some kind of humble pie spin-off, but the bottom line is it builds character to be able to do it. And life has a lot of that, so they might as well learn it now. They'll be happier for it, too. They all are.

I worked with a high school kid once who kept getting subpar grades and was obviously intelligent. I warned this kid, for at least two semesters that if they tanked their grades again I'd see to it they got grounded. Sure enough, crappy grades. Sure enough, I called the mom in and I laid out a plan: a full semester of no socializing, no phone, no internet…no nothin'. The kid immediately mentioned a birthday party for a close friend that was in two days. The mom wavered. I said, "Yeah, no. You won't be going." The kid was crushed...and got over it. The semester progressed, and the kid actually did their own adherence to the "grounding" by the near end of the semester. Why? Because kids crave boundaries – they don't like them, but they sense they need them. And they don't have to like them, railing against rules is part of their job as a teen, they do have to follow them, or face more consequences. So how did it turn out? That kid got straight A's the last three semesters in a row of high school. Then they went on to a big university and rocked it – four B's and all the rest A's in all of college. The graduation ceremony is this month. I'm incredibly proud.

Don't be a F**kin Narcissist

I don't mean narcissist in the way it's used in everyday layperson's terms. Man, narcissism is an infinitely complex psychological disorder that people really suffer from, and society has reduced all that into it being just a synonym for "asshole." I hate that. (I'm going do something about that in my *next* book). No, when I instruct *you* in this context, what I mean is sometimes, as a parent, you gotta do shit you hate for the benefit of your kid. You have to teach them the things they need to know in order to be successful and happy in the world at large. And, like it or not, that means sometimes *you* need to be the "bad guy." You are *not* your kid's friend. They have friends, and they're their own age. You're too old to be their friend. They don't want old friends.

And why would you want a friend that young? That's weird. When I hear someone say that they're their kid's friend, I wanna puke. All I hear in that is, "I suffer from such a pervasive feeling of inadequacy that I don't even step in and discipline my kid when they're fucking up because I'm so fragile in who I am, I need everyone – including my kid – to think I'm a Good Guy, and my needs come before the well-being of the person I brought into the world and am responsible for." Gross. *Gross!*

I hope that you can see how destructive that is. It's not about *you*. You made a person, so you accepted the job of doing what best for *them*, even when it's hard for *you*. You being uncomfortable is irrelevant. Suck it up. It's your kid. Do the right thing. And if you are co-parenting, it is so, *so* important to go at this whole plan as a *united front*. Whatever adults are in charge of your kid's health and well-being, get them on board with your new plan. Separate houses, your parent that lives with you, teachers, shrinks, *everybody*. As the kid's clinician, I can only support your consequences if you *have* consequences. I love few things more than laughing at a kid when they complain to me that they snuck out or something, got caught, and now can't do something they want to do because their parents are so mean, and don't I think that's so unfair? No! I think it's funny. I think your parents are doing their goddamn job! And, frankly, I'm surprised you would come in here with me and try and float that sad-faced, sorry-ass plea for validation. It's the perfect set-up for me to drop one of my famous lines: "You want some cheese with that whine?" Aaaah, classic

Dr. Kelly stuff. And then my making fun of them in that moment tells them:

1. I'm not an idiot
2. I totally agree with their parents' decision
3. I think their parents' decision is *for them* (the kid) and keeping them safe
4. I believe they have the self-esteem, ego-strength, and resilience to handle a sick burn like the classic I just laid down

CHAPTER 11
ROAMING AROUND IN THE DARK.... DYS-REGULATED (DBT TERM)

So, at this point you may or may not understand that this problem, your kid cutting themselves, is *way* too big a thing for you to handle without help. And why *wouldn't* it be!? Why our society allows us all to walk around without an emotional education is beyond me. When all of us are humans, and all humans experience emotions, you would think we would want to know all about emotions: What they are, how to identify and name them, how they feel in our bodies, what to *do* when we have them, and on and on. Psychology, the science of human emotions and behavior is, for some reason, not something we value getting to know. It's so practical in our everyday lives, I don't

get why it's still such a mystery to most. I have theories.
I think emotions scare people because sometimes they
are powerful. I think in a male-dominated society, anything generalized as female isn't seen as powerful – which
contradicts why people would be scared of them, then…
hmmmm. Does that translate into females are powerful
and if we keep people ignorant of emotions we can keep
females from ruling the world!? A discussion for another
day.

Point is, I believe it is truly no fault of yours that you
had no idea how to handle your kid's cutting before you
opened this book. I mean it. Cutting is a weird, secret,
scary, widely misunderstood behavior, even by most professionals in the field of mental health. Until we start
teaching children about their emotions in school, I don't
see how we will eliminate crises like the one you're in
now. But now you know there *is* help out there. You'll
have to sift through the drones and lemmings of *any* pro-
fession, but you have read this book so you know a helluva lot more about your kid's problem than you once
did. So, kudos to you. That was a seriously brave step –
and you *know* I didn't sugar-coat it to go down easy! But
you're here. And you have the *real*-deal information now.
The shit very few people would ever tell you. So what are
you going to do now?

I would think, with the new knowledge and confidence you have because of what you just read, that you
might be tempted to just try this on your own. No. No.
A thousand times no. You *do* know more now than the
vast majority of people. But untreated – and I mean *by* a

professional – you are still out of your depth. I have given you some commonalities of kids that engage in cutting behaviors, but it remains true that everyone is different. And that variability, and you without a license, means the treatment plan still needs to include someone qualified to give treatment. For something as serious as cutting and, really, *all* self-harm behaviors, that means someone with training. There are a lot of things that went off the rails for someone who resorts to hurting themselves on purpose as a way to cope. That does *not* change overnight, and, in fact, tends to get worse without proper, effective treatment. You don't want your kid to decompensate even more. I don't want your kid to decompensate even more. And without professional help that's what the numbers tell us will happen. You have a shot, right now, to take swift and immediate action. You now have a clear idea what the problem *is* so you can *do* something about it.

You don't know where this goes from here if you "go possum" on this, but I do. You'll spend tens of thousands of dollars on a wilderness program, and/or a therapeutic boarding school, and/or an inpatient rehab facility, and/or legal fees, and/or your kid is still/back living with you in their thirties, etc. You're going to spend some money and time on this, so why not get the most bang for your buck *now?* I know therapy is expensive, and, newsflash, your kid may need to start at twice a week *and* take a DBT class. And though you may see some positive results right away, these behaviors took years to develop and will take some time to undo. And I don't want you to start this process and then get scared or impatient and mood-dependently decide that's "good enough." I really can't tell you how heartbreaking it is to watch parents yank their kids from working with me at the first glimmers of progress, only to have them come back a couple years later with a huge shitstorm that they now want me to "solve." I'm good, but I'm not a friggin' miracle-worker (though I *was* in that high school production). Bottom line is, if you attack this problem now, blinders off and big girl/boy panties on, you really have a shot at getting your kid's life on a path that can be even better than before all this mess. I know you can do it. I know you can.

CHAPTER 12
AT THE END OF
THE DAY...

———————————

It is my sincere wish and belief that you will have such an effective and successful structure in place to deal with the mood-dependent (mess-making) decisions your kid has made that you, as parents, will feel confident in immediately spotting and correcting any future behaviors that your kid may engage in that may hurt them or their future happiness. Let's just go over how you learned to do this:

1. Acknowledge your own feelings about finding out your kid is cutting: fear, guilt, worry, sadness, regret, etc. And whatever feelings you feel, they are valid, so validate them – even naming them is a form of validation. The *thoughts* you have that are derived from these feelings may or may not be valid, but we can't even assess that until you have regulated all your emotions. Then, we can remember you are not the only one whose kid cuts themselves and there *is* help out there.

2. Remember that cutting is a form of self-medicating like any other form of self-medication: drinking, drugs, shopping, over-working, binge-eating, etc. Most humans engage or have engaged in some form of avoiding their intense and negative feelings and coping tools can be taught to replace these current unhealthy coping mechanisms.

3. There are probably some things that are unknown to you causing distress in your kid that are contributing to their cutting behavior. You need to talk and then listen to your kid and find out what those things *are*. Put yourself in their shoes and think of how hard it would be for you to be their age in the world today. What do you imagine you would struggle with? Ask them what struggles are unique to *them*. Have the courage to ask your kid what they are angry about and then listen to them when they answer…even if you are part of it. Know how lucky you are for them to even open up to you.

4. Know that, depending on the kid, there are often options other than psychotropic medications. You'll want to assess with professionals what the options are for your kid and pick the best one. Medications may end up being one tool for helping your kid's recovery, but they are likely not the only option. Most kids who hurt themselves on purpose need to talk.

5. You now know that things probably are gonna get pretty bumpy before they level out. Keep

going! They *will* level out. Effective communication helps any emotionally charged situation, and if you need parenting help it's out there, so go get it.

6. It is supremely important to shop around to get the right professional to work with your kid. You don't want someone who just says smart words. You want a clinician who *listens* and *connects* with your kid. Set up lots of appointments and ask your kid who they connected with and why – then listen to their answer. When they pick, hold them to it. They're going to get help – end of story. This is too serious not to.

7. You now have a detailed plan to put in place in your home. This plan will make you feel informed and in control as parents, and will make your kid(s) feel secure knowing what to expect in all circumstances involving your family's values and expectations. You will feel confident handling disciplinary situations with firmness and compassion, knowing that boundaries are the thing that make kids feel safe.

The very best of luck to you and your family. I have seen lots and lots of kids emerge from a very similar situation to the hell your kid's in now – and they have become smart, confident, silly, articulate, creative, thoughtful, joyful leaders in their communities. They love and like themselves, and it shows! I am so proud of all of them, and I know your kid can be just like them.

ACKNOWLEDGEMENTS

To the Author Incubator team: Special thanks again to Angela Lauria, CEO & Founder of The Author Incubator for being a one-of-a-kind warrior-goddess of love and change. To my Developmental Editor Mehrina Asif and Managing Editor, Moriah Howell, thanks for corralling me just enough, but not too much. Many more thanks to everyone else at TAI, but especially Aicha Bascaro, and Tami Stackelhouse.

And sincere thanks to all the people that have trusted me with their most intimate moments, thoughts, and feelings. I have trouble putting into words the joy I feel when we do the work together. It has been my privilege and my pleasure...even the rough days.

~ Best. Job. Ever. ~

ABOUT
THE AUTHOR

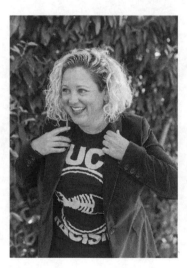

Dr. J.J. Kelly is a licensed clinical psychologist who specializes in Teens & Young Adults, Dialectical Behavior Therapy (DBT), and Joy. Dr. Kelly has practiced in Berkeley, California, for the last fifteen years, though she was born in the Midwest. She started her current practice with a deep intentionality around intersection and inclusion.

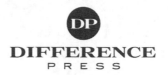

ABOUT
DIFFERENCE PRESS

Difference Press is the exclusive publishing arm of The Author Incubator, an educational company for entrepreneurs – including life coaches, healers, consultants, and community leaders – looking for a comprehensive solution to get their books written, published, and promoted. Its founder, Dr. Angela Lauria, has been bringing to life the literary ventures of hundreds of authors-in-transformation since 1994.

A boutique-style self-publishing service for clients of The Author Incubator, Difference Press boasts a fair and easy-to-understand profit structure, low-priced author copies, and author-friendly contract terms. Most importantly, all of our #incubatedauthors maintain ownership of their copyright at all times.

Let's Start a Movement with Your Message

In a market where hundreds of thousands of books are published every year and are never heard from again,

The Author Incubator is different. Not only do all Difference Press books reach Amazon bestseller status, but all of our authors are actively changing lives and making a difference.

Since launching in 2013, we've served over 500 authors who came to us with an idea for a book and were able to write it and get it self-published in less than 6 months. In addition, more than 100 of those books were picked up by traditional publishers and are now available in bookstores. We do this by selecting the highest quality and highest potential applicants for our future programs.

Our program doesn't only teach you how to write a book – our team of coaches, developmental editors, copy editors, art directors, and marketing experts incubate you from having a book idea to being a published, bestselling author, ensuring that the book you create can actually make a difference in the world. Then we give you the training you need to use your book to make the difference in the world, or to create a business out of serving your readers.

Are You Ready to Make a Difference?

You've seen other people make a difference with a book. Now it's your turn. If you are ready to stop watching and start taking massive action, go to http://theauthorincubator.com/apply/.

"Yes, I'm ready!"

OTHER BOOKS BY DIFFERENCE PRESS

---

*Reverse Button™: Learn What the Doctors Aren't Telling You,
Avoid Back Surgery, and Get Your Full Life Back*
by Abby Beauchamp

*Never Too Late for Love: The Successful Woman's Guide to
Online Dating in the Second Half of Life*
by Joan Bragar, EdD

Stronger Together: My MS Story
by Chloe Cohen

Yogini's Dilemma: To Be, or Not to Be, a Yoga Teacher?
by Nicole A. Grant

*Come Alive: Find Your Passion, Change Your Life, Change the
World!* by Jodi Hadsell

*Meant For More: Stop Secretly Struggling and Become
a Force to Be Reckoned With*
by Mia Hewett

Lord, Please Save My Marriage: A Christian Woman's Guide to Thrive, Despite Her Husband's Drunken Rants
by Christine Lennard

If I'm so Zen, Why Is My Hair Falling Out?: How Past Trauma and Anxiety Manifest in the Physical Body
by Amanda Lera

Heal Your Trauma, Heal Your Marriage: 7 Steps to Root, Rebound, and Rise
by Dr. Cheri L. McDonald

WELCOME to the Next Level: 3 Secrets to Become Unstuck, Take Action, and Rise Higher in Your Career
by Sonya L. Sigler

Embrace Your Psychic Gifts: The Guide to Spiritual Awakening
by Deborah Sudarsky

Leverage: The Guide to End Your Binge Eating
by Linda Vang

Under the Sleeve: Find Help for Your Child Who Is Cutting
by Dr. Stacey Winters

THANK YOU!

Thanks for putting this book to good use. If you'd like to stay connected, please email through **drjjkelly.com** for bonus materials.